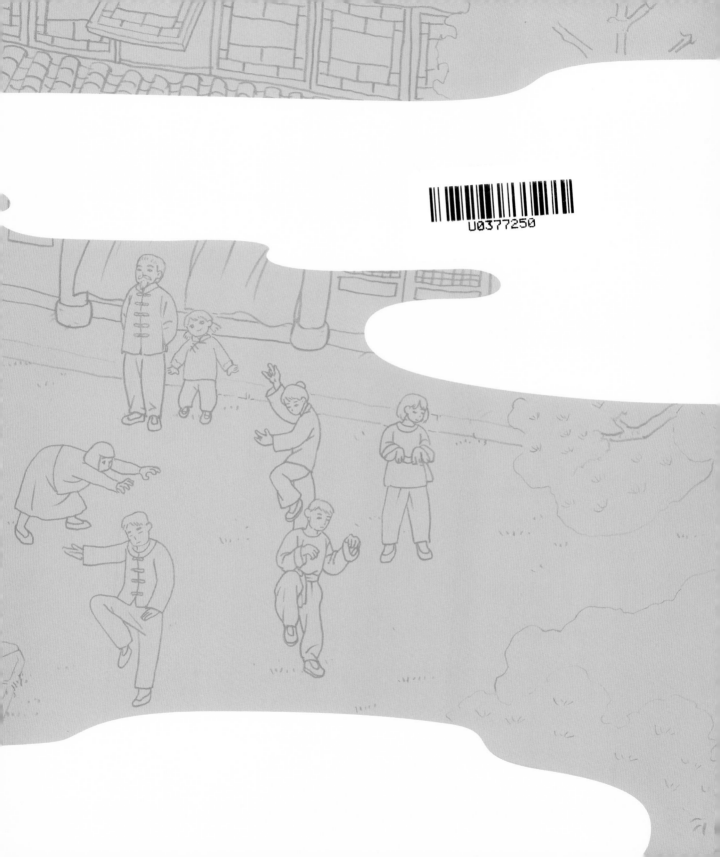

走进中医治未病

Traditional Chinese Medicine on Preventive Treatment

编委会名单

主　编　郁东海　范春香

副主编　都乐亦　张　莉　卢江虹

绘　画　落小山　周　全

翻　译　朴永镇　贾　静

编　委　（按姓氏笔画排序）

王　琦　王　慧　卢江虹　齐佳龙　花迎雪

李鹏帆　杨燕婷　沈　丽　张　莉　范春香

郁东海　赵　玫　胡晓萍　胡新民　都乐亦

徐森华　曾艺鹏　解雨彤

复旦大學出版社

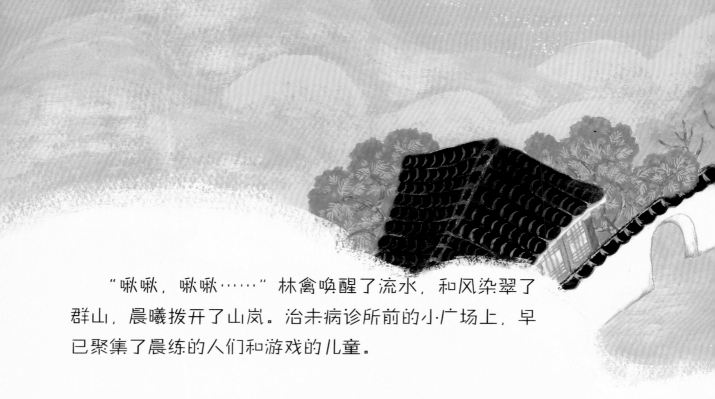

　　"啾啾，啾啾⋯⋯"林禽唤醒了流水，和风染翠了群山，晨曦拨开了山岚。治未病诊所前的小广场上，早已聚集了晨练的人们和游戏的儿童。

"Chirp, chirp, chirp …" Forest birds awakened the stream, a gentle breeze dyed the mountains green, and the morning sun dispersed the mist. Morning walkers and children playing games had already gathered in the small square in front of the Preventative Medicine Clinic.

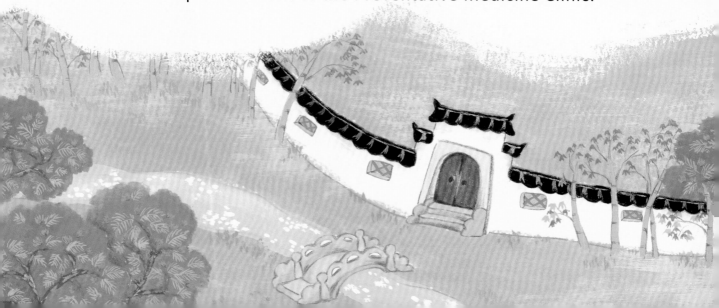

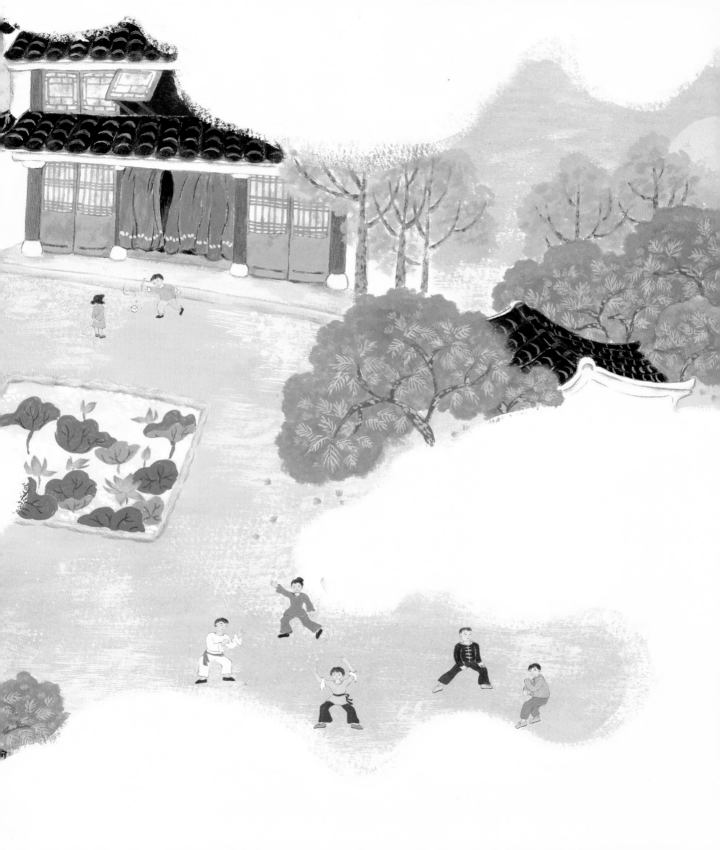

未病先防　Prevention Before Disease Onset

顺应节气

这天是端午节。

小朋友们吃起了粽子、鸭蛋。诊所里的人从深山觅来草药，专方配制成香囊，闻着使人通体舒泰；又在门上挂起菖蒲，驱蛇蝎、避蚊虫。

Living with the Seasons

It was the Dragon Boat Festival.

The children enjoyed rice dumplings (*Zongzi*) and duck eggs. The practitioners of the clinic gathered herbs from the mountains and made them into sachet bags (known as "*Xiangnang*") with a soothing aroma. Additionally, they hung calamus leaves on the door to repel snakes, scorpions, and mosquitoes.

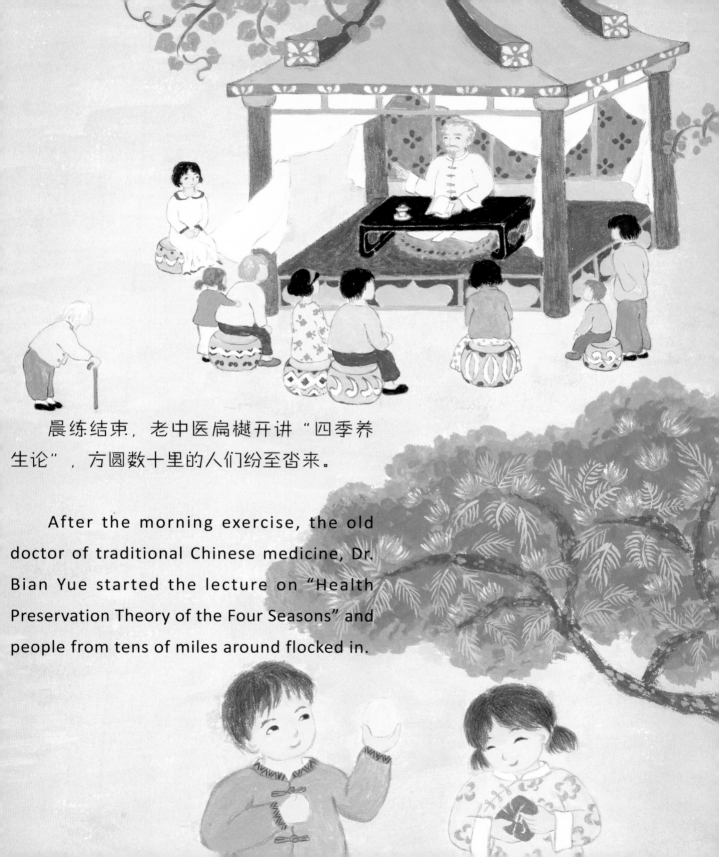

　　晨练结束，老中医扁樾开讲"四季养生论"，方圆数十里的人们纷至沓来。

After the morning exercise, the old doctor of traditional Chinese medicine, Dr. Bian Yue started the lecture on "Health Preservation Theory of the Four Seasons" and people from tens of miles around flocked in.

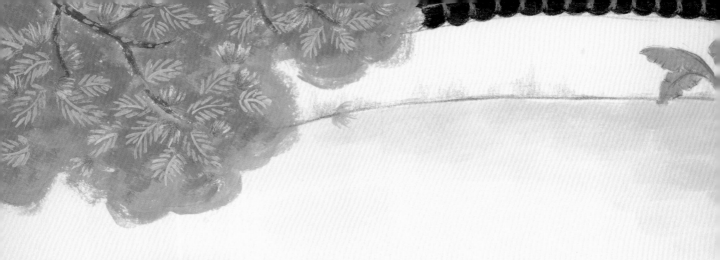

小儿增高

　　一位母亲领着年已十三、身形却尚如童子的少年前来就医。一番望闻问切后，老中医让自己的孙女巧儿领少年在诊所暂住。

　　不长个的原因很多，包括先天不足、后天失养，需要综合考虑。

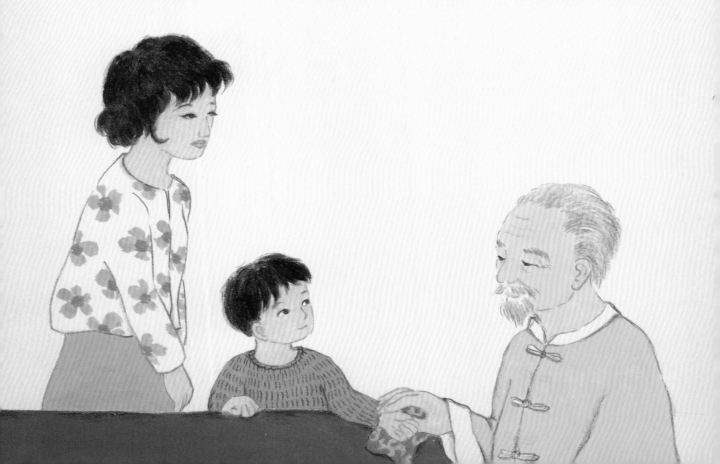

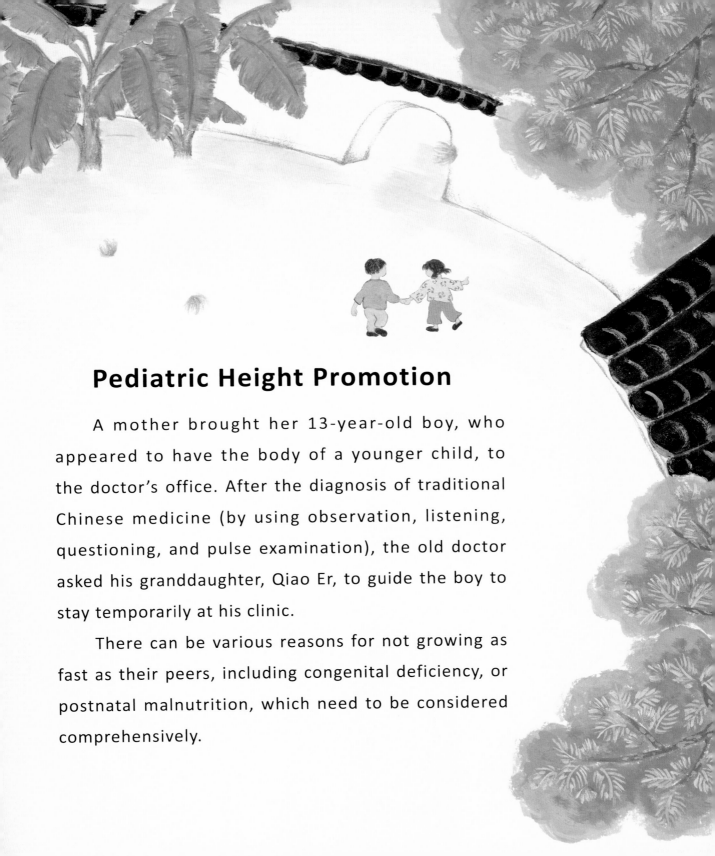

Pediatric Height Promotion

A mother brought her 13-year-old boy, who appeared to have the body of a younger child, to the doctor's office. After the diagnosis of traditional Chinese medicine (by using observation, listening, questioning, and pulse examination), the old doctor asked his granddaughter, Qiao Er, to guide the boy to stay temporarily at his clinic.

There can be various reasons for not growing as fast as their peers, including congenital deficiency, or postnatal malnutrition, which need to be considered comprehensively.

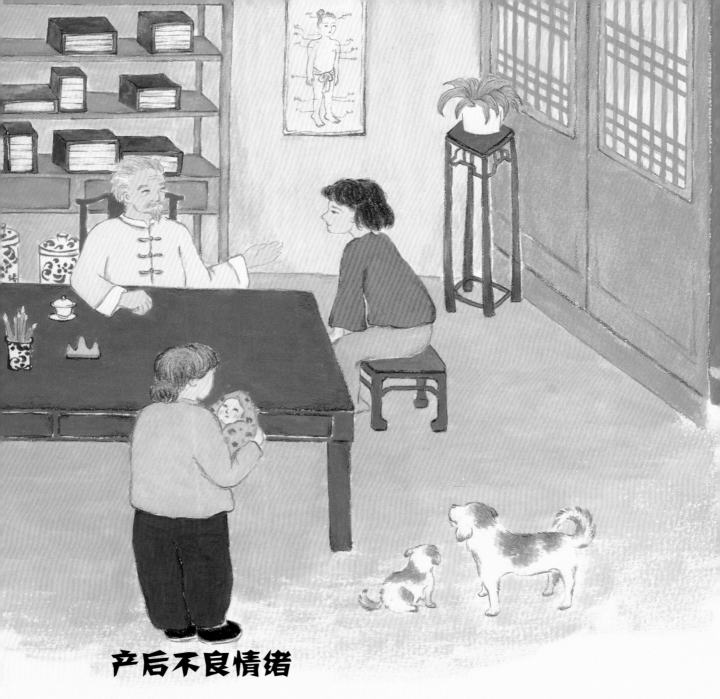

产后不良情绪

　　女子在月子期间会经常感到沮丧、烦躁、疲惫，仿佛万念俱灰。年轻妈妈晓晴望着老中医，一脸沮丧。

　　育儿压力、脱离人际交往导致她肝气郁结、心神失养，这种现象很普遍。老中医开出方子，嘱咐她按时服药。

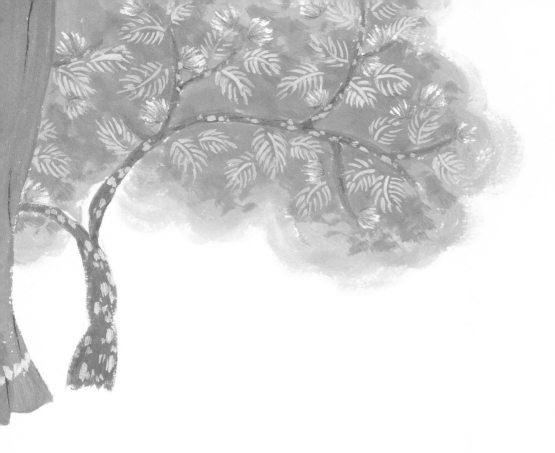

Postpartum Adverse Emotions

The postpartum period of woman is often characterized by depression, irritability, exhaustion, and a sense of apathy. Xiao Qing, the young mother, gazed at the old doctor with a frustrated expression.

The woman's parenting stress and lack of socialization had led to her liver *qi* stagnation and her heart-mind failing to be nourished, which is very common nowadays. The old doctor prescribed a formula and told her to take it on time.

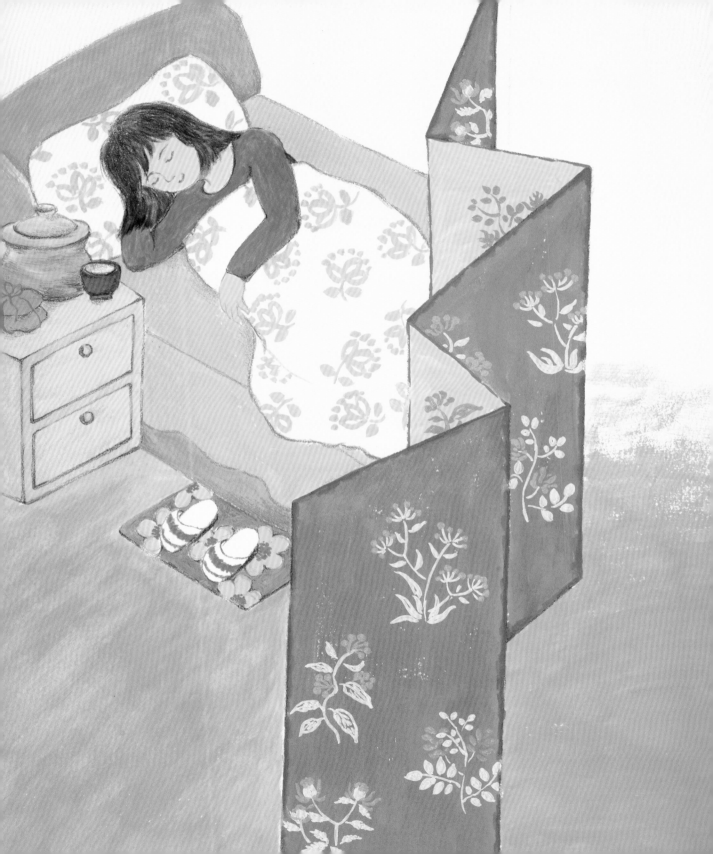

更年期不适状态

刚从教师岗位退休的雅君最近常常心烦意乱、茶饭不思、多梦易醒、潮热盗汗。

Menopausal Discomfort State

Recently, Ya Jun, who had just retired from teaching, suffered from restlessness, poor appetite, dream-disturbed sleep, tidal fever and night sweats.

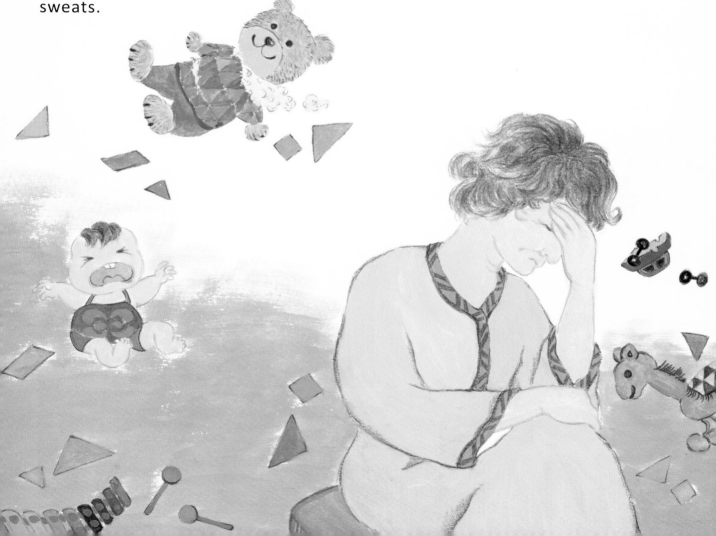

老中医开了中成药，教她有空做一些简单的穴位按摩。

The old doctor prescribed Chinese patent medicines and recommended her to do some basic acupressure massage at her leisure.

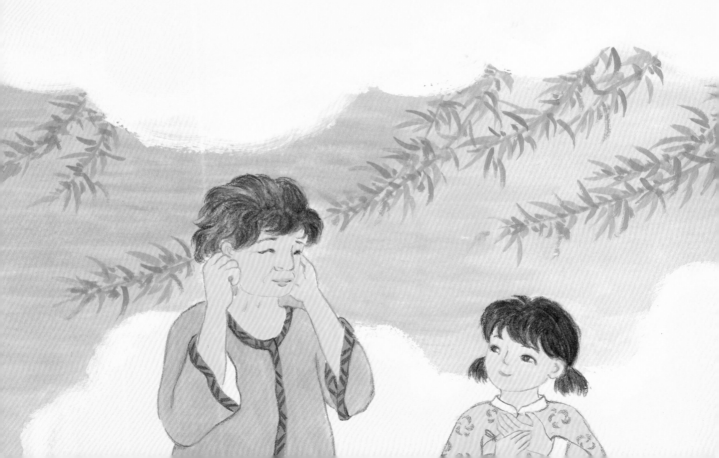

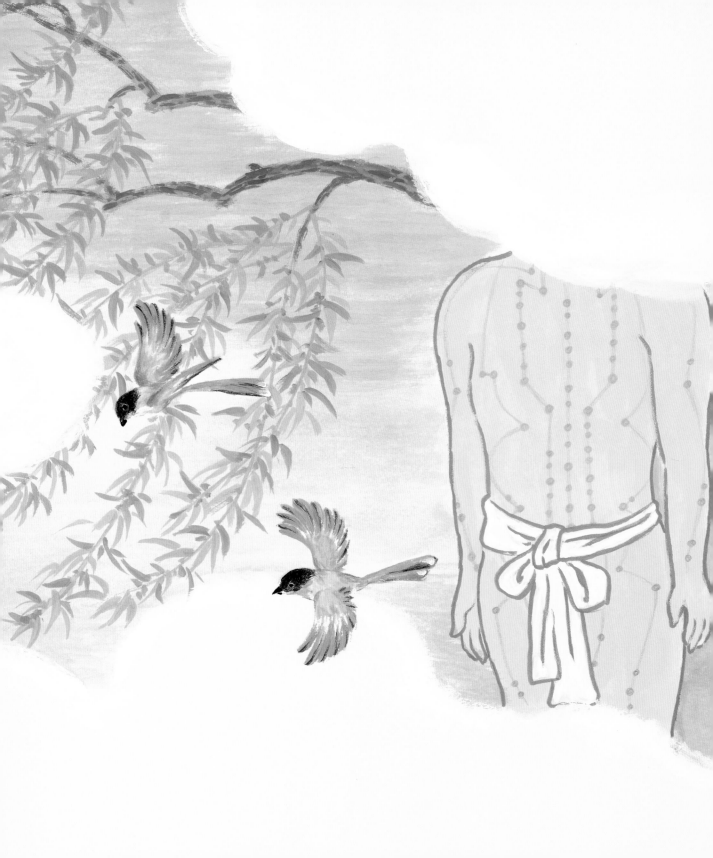

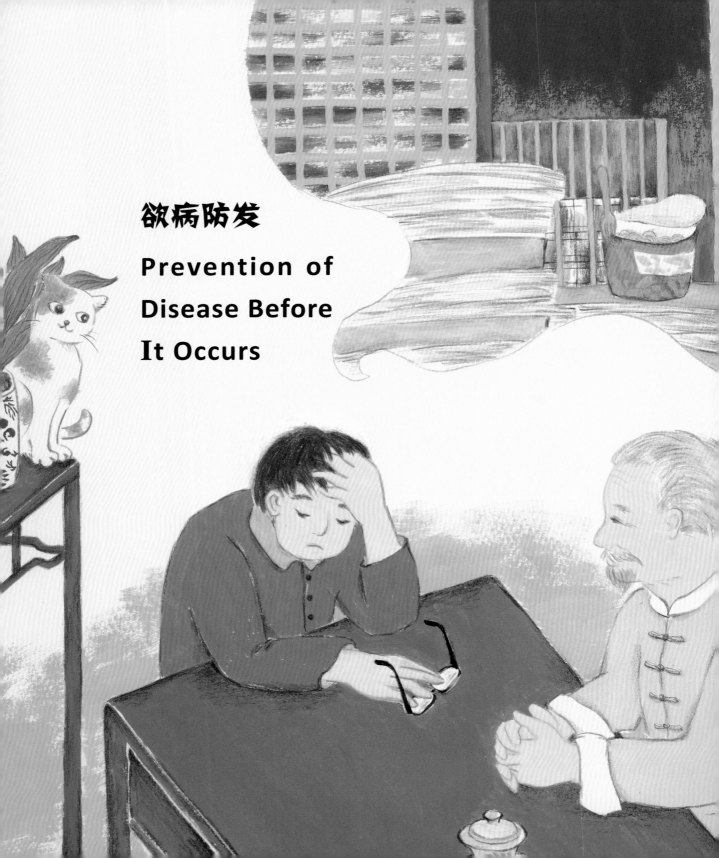

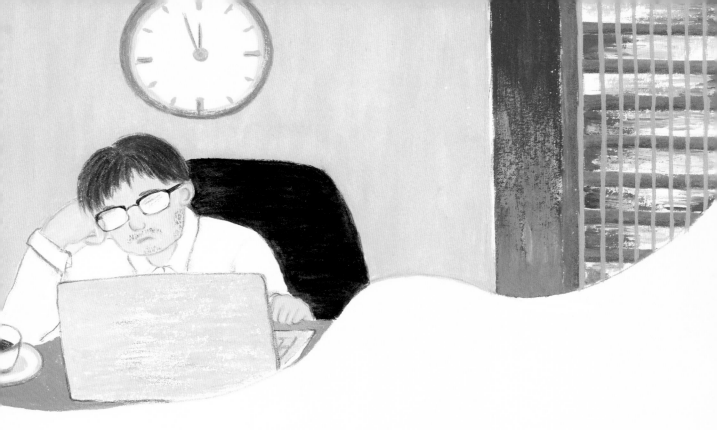

上班族的烦恼

白天犯困、晚上失眠，记忆力下降，注意力不集中，上班族小·李坐在老中医面前，满脸颓丧。

Trouble with Commuters

Mr. Li, an office worker, sat in front of the old doctor with a depressed face. He had experienced daytime sleepiness, nighttime insomnia, poor memory and lack of concentration recently.

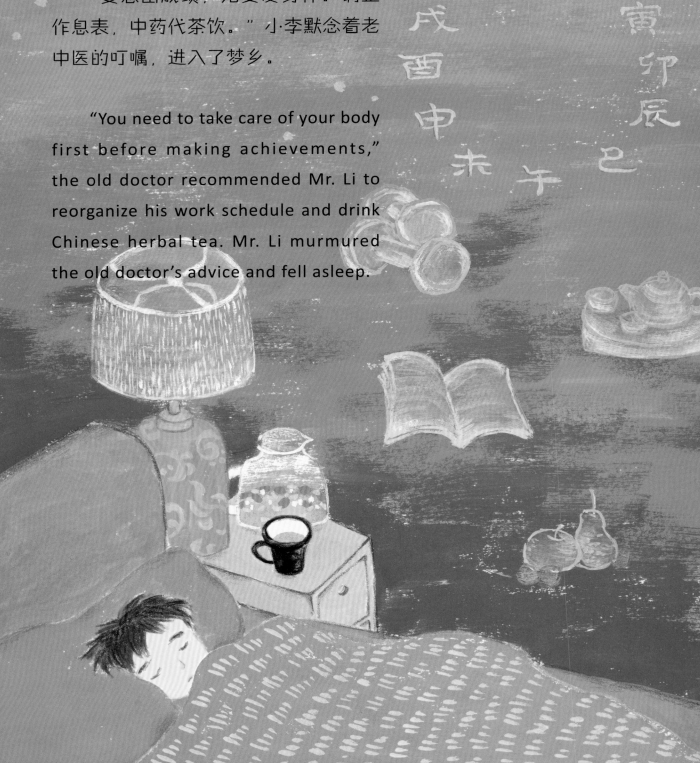

"要想出成绩，先要爱身体。调整作息表，中药代茶饮。"小李默念着老中医的叮嘱，进入了梦乡。

"You need to take care of your body first before making achievements," the old doctor recommended Mr. Li to reorganize his work schedule and drink Chinese herbal tea. Mr. Li murmured the old doctor's advice and fell asleep.

子 丑 寅 卯 辰 巳 午 未 申 酉 戌 亥

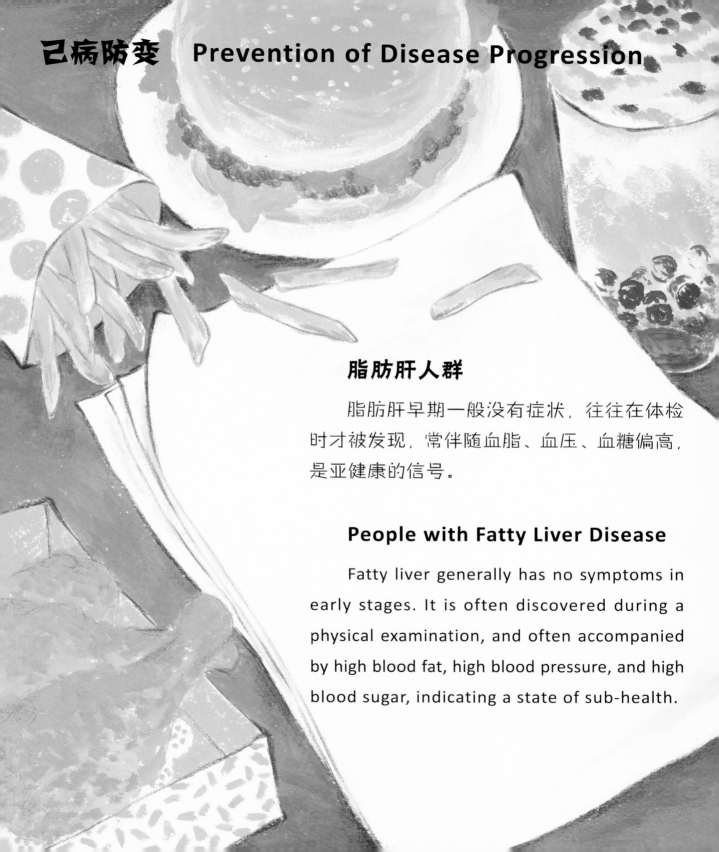

脂肪肝人群

脂肪肝早期一般没有症状，往往在体检时才被发现，常伴随血脂、血压、血糖偏高，是亚健康的信号。

People with Fatty Liver Disease

Fatty liver generally has no symptoms in early stages. It is often discovered during a physical examination, and often accompanied by high blood fat, high blood pressure, and high blood sugar, indicating a state of sub-health.

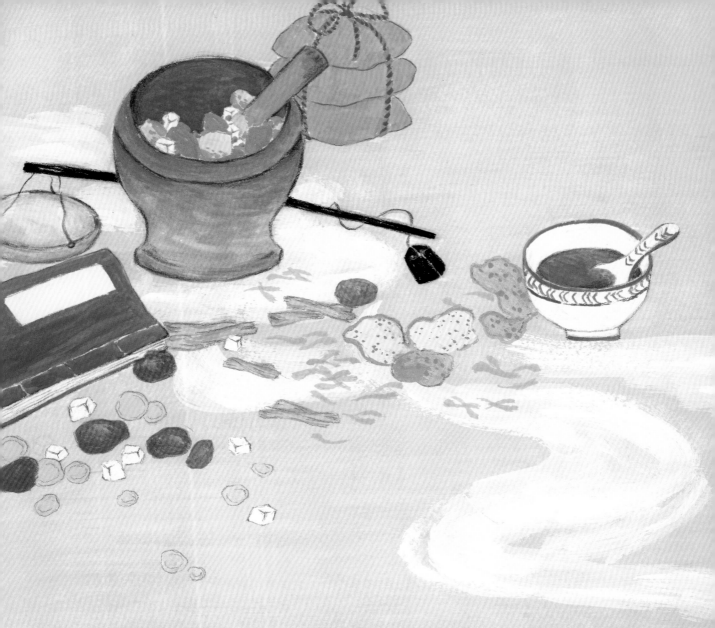

饮食清淡、适度锻炼、调适情志、辅以方药，便能回归健康。

Adopting a light diet, engaging in moderate exercises, regulating emotions, and being supplemented with Chinese herbal formulas will contribute to restoring health.

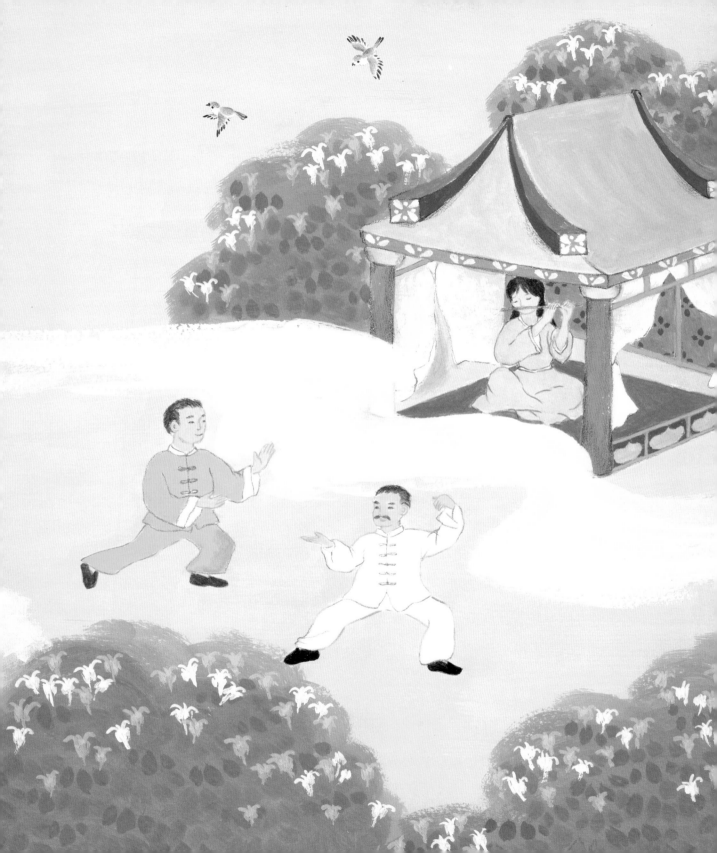

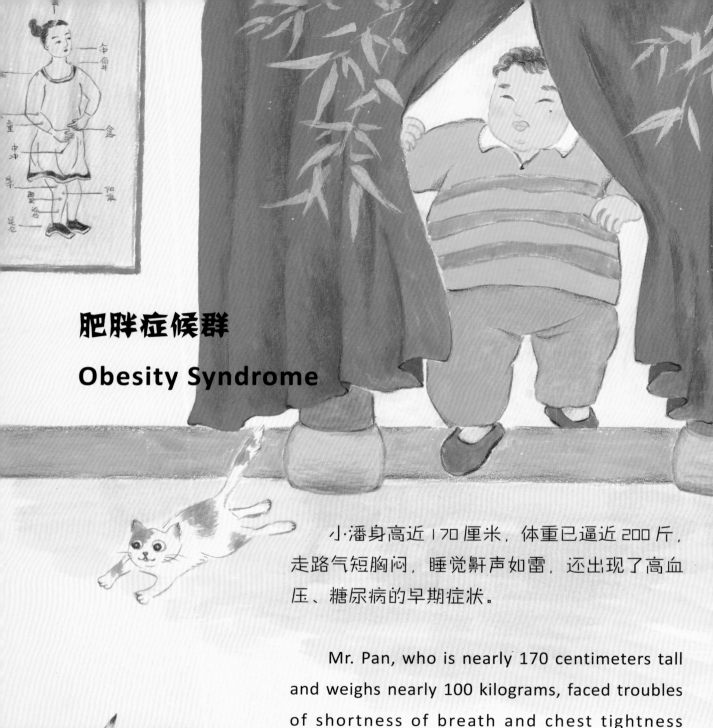

肥胖症候群
Obesity Syndrome

小·潘身高近170厘米，体重已逼近200斤，走路气短胸闷，睡觉鼾声如雷，还出现了高血压、糖尿病的早期症状。

Mr. Pan, who is nearly 170 centimeters tall and weighs nearly 100 kilograms, faced troubles of shortness of breath and chest tightness while walking. He also experienced loud snoring during sleep, and early signs of hypertension and diabetes had begun to appear.

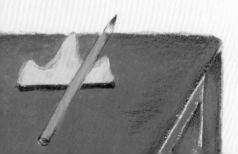

肥胖问题解决了，其他自然能好转。老中医开出了方药、药膳，并配合理疗，对症下药、多管齐下。

Resolving the obesity problem is crucial, as it could positively impact other health aspects. The old doctor prescribed Chinese herbal formulas, medicinal diets, and combined with physical therapy, taking a symptomatic and multi-faceted approach.

病后防复 Prevention of Recurrence After Disease

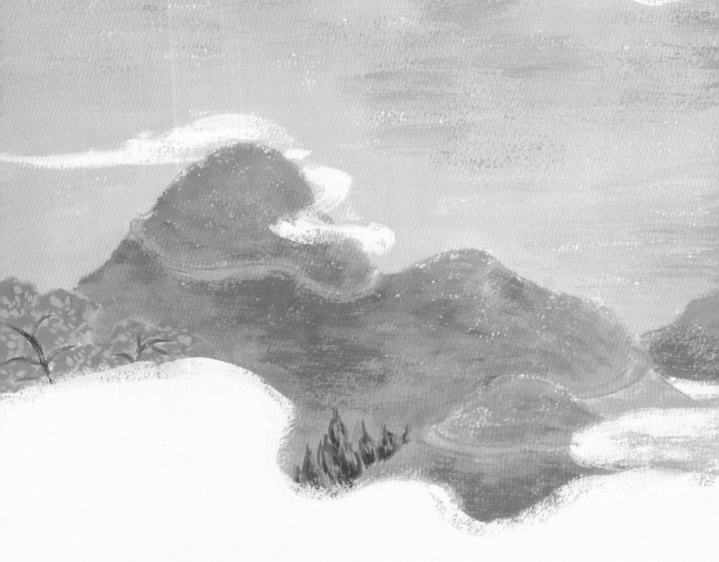

脑卒中患者

"叮铃铃……"在一阵急促的电话铃声召唤下，老中医坐上了越野车，沿着逶迤山路，穿越层峦叠嶂，直奔一位脑卒中患者家中。

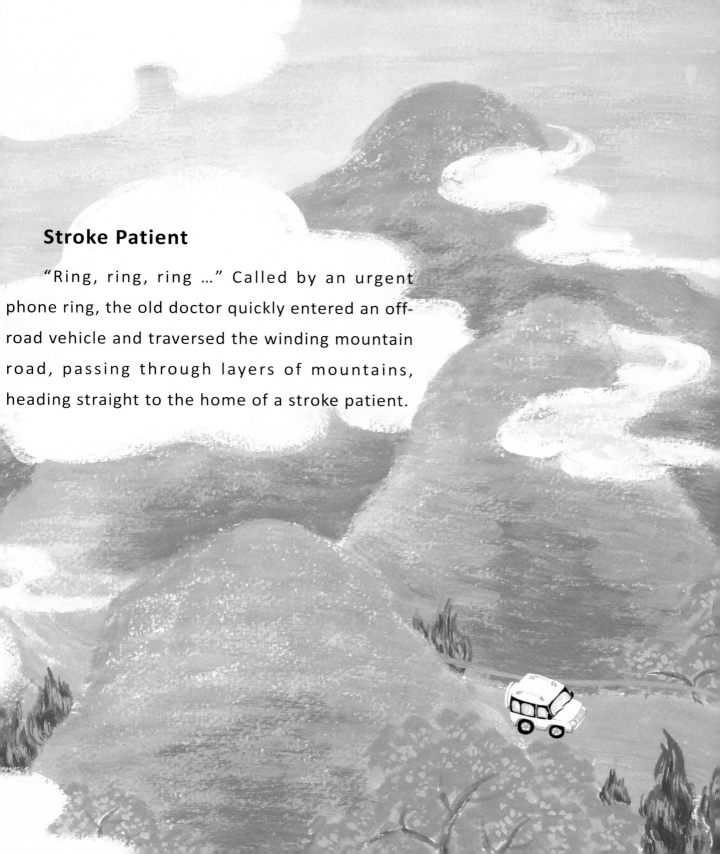

Stroke Patient

"Ring, ring, ring …" Called by an urgent phone ring, the old doctor quickly entered an off-road vehicle and traversed the winding mountain road, passing through layers of mountains, heading straight to the home of a stroke patient.

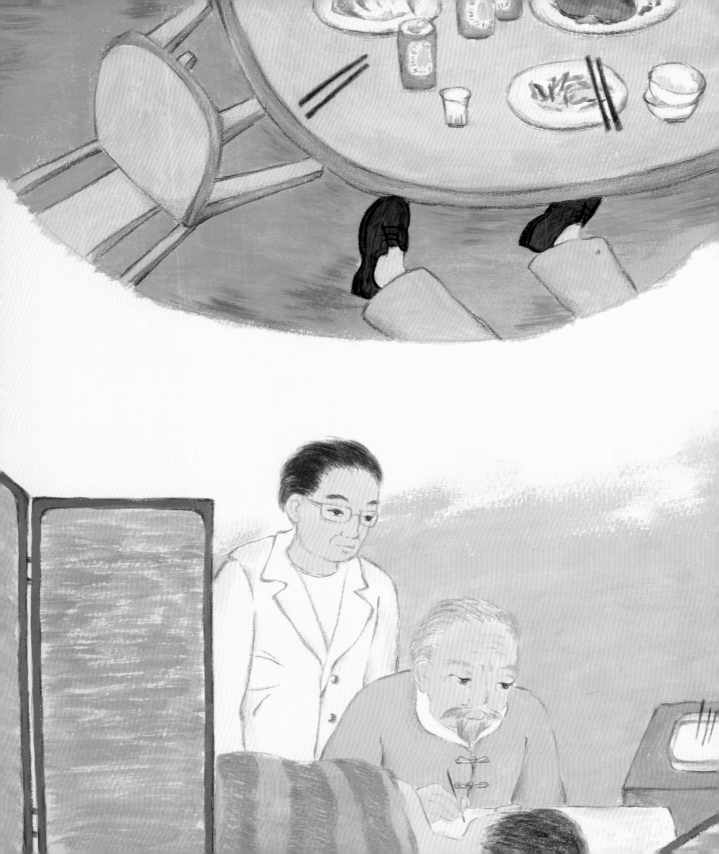

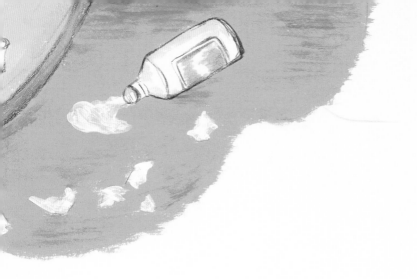

这位昨晚还在应酬的中年男子，此刻刚被抢救回来，但仍处于偏瘫麻木中，老中医打开针灸包，开始治疗。

The middle-aged man who had attended the dinner party last night was just resuscitated, but he was still experiencing hemiplegic numbness. The old doctor opened his acupuncture bag and started the treatment.

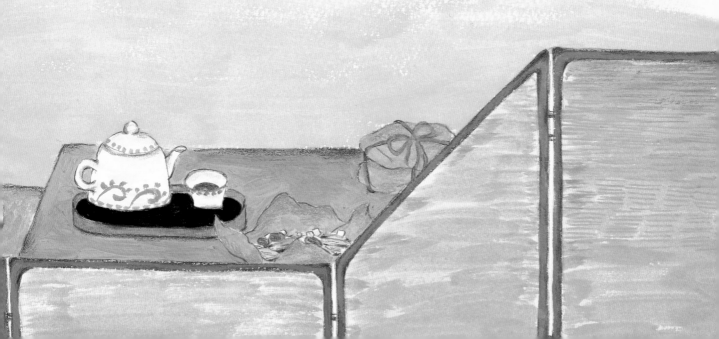

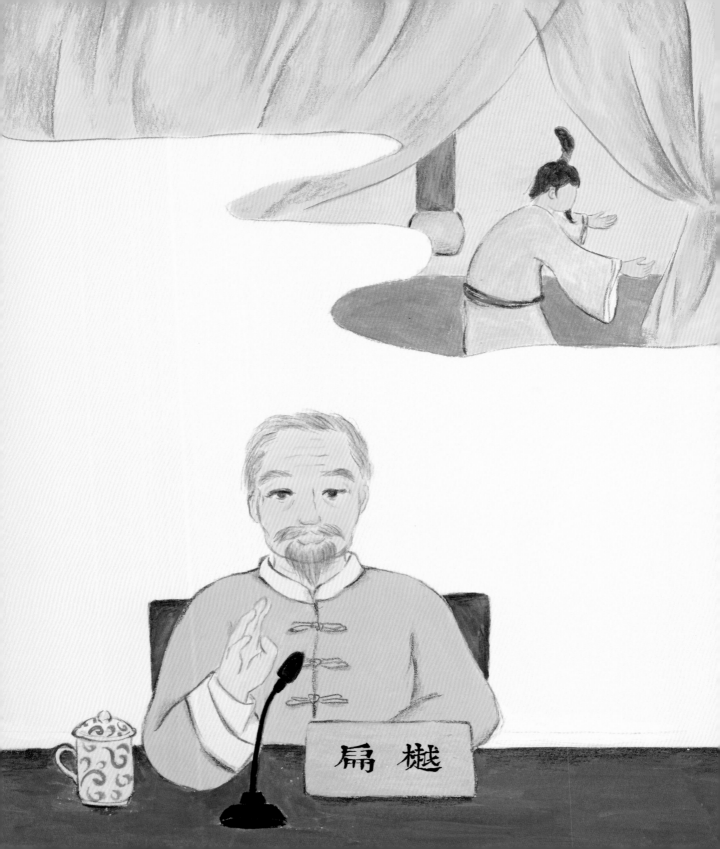

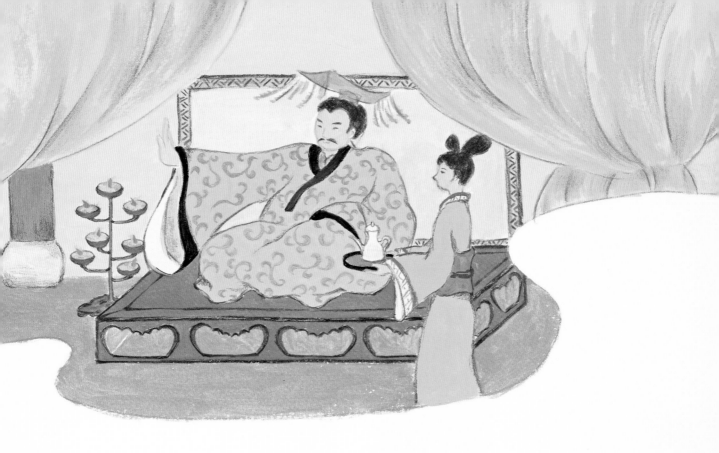

　　一年一度的“治未病学术研讨会”上，老中医谈到扁鹊见蔡桓公的故事，桓公因讳疾忌医，导致“未病”终不可医。

At the annual "Symposium on Preventive Treatment of Disease", the old doctor talked about the story of the renowned Chinese physician Bian Que meeting Duke Cai Huan. In the story, Duke Cai Huan hid his disease instead of seeking medical care, and in the end, he passed away without receiving timely medical care.

《黄帝内经》云："上工治未病。"传统中医学，法天地自然，顺四时之变，维阴平阳秘，保心志闲舒。如今人们关注亚健康概念，正是治未病大显身手的好时候。

The *Huangdi Neijing (Inner Canon of Yellow Emperor)* says, "The superior doctor prevents sickness." In traditional Chinese medicine theory, we should strive to follow the rules of nature and live in accordance with the changing seasons, maintaining harmony between *yin* and *yang* and cultivating peace of mind. Nowadays people pay attention to the concept of sub-health, which is a good time that preventive treatment of disease can play its full role.

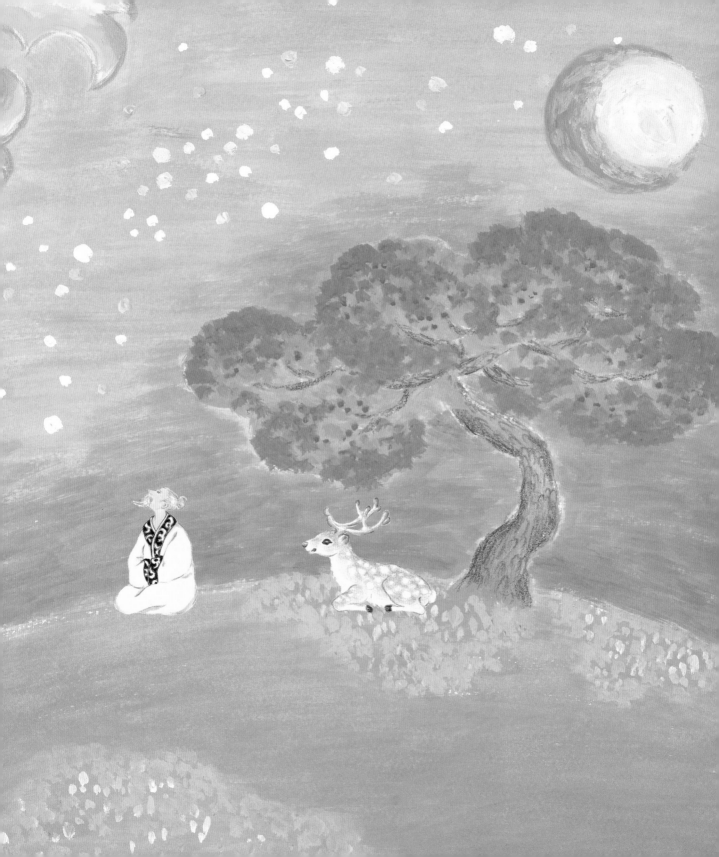

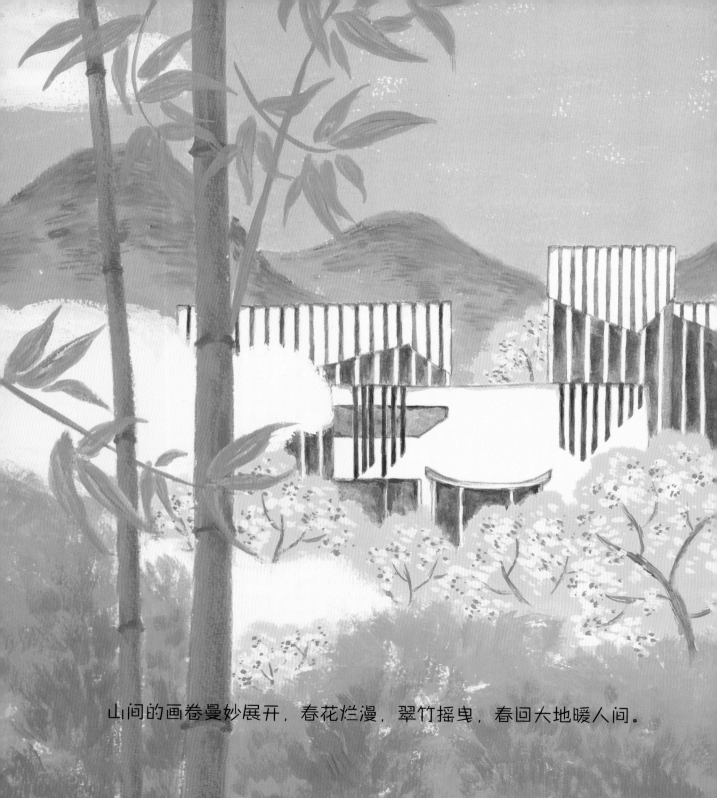

山间的画卷曼妙展开，春花烂漫，翠竹摇曳，春回大地暖人间。

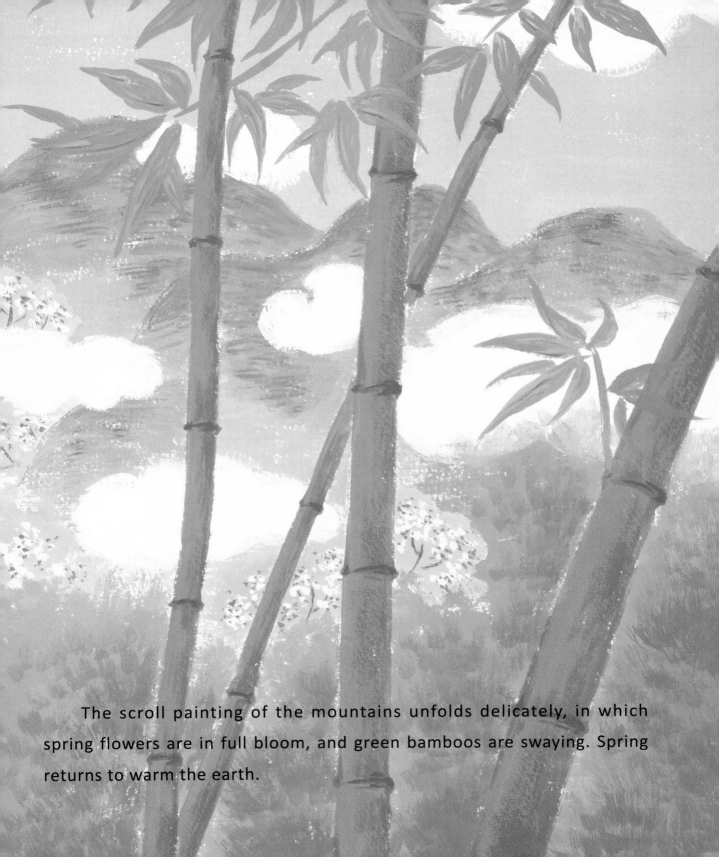

The scroll painting of the mountains unfolds delicately, in which spring flowers are in full bloom, and green bamboos are swaying. Spring returns to warm the earth.

图书在版编目(CIP)数据

走进中医治未病/郁东海,范春香主编;落小山,周全绘画;朴永镇,贾静翻译.—上海:复旦大学出版社,2024.1
ISBN 978-7-309-17161-7

Ⅰ.①走⋯ Ⅱ.①郁⋯ ②范⋯ ③落⋯ ④周⋯ ⑤朴⋯ ⑥贾⋯ Ⅲ.①中医学-预防医学
Ⅳ.①R211

中国国家版本馆 CIP 数据核字(2024)第 000783 号

走进中医治未病

郁东海　范春香　主编
落小山　周　全　绘画
朴永镇　贾　静　翻译
责任编辑/张　怡

复旦大学出版社有限公司出版发行
上海市国权路 579 号　邮编:200433
网址:fupnet@ fudanpress.com　http://www.fudanpress.com
门市零售:86-21-65102580　团体订购:86-21-65104505
出版部电话:86-21-65642845
上海雅昌艺术印刷有限公司

开本 889 毫米×1194 毫米　1/20　印张 2　字数 30 千字
2024 年 1 月第 1 版
2024 年 1 月第 1 版第 1 次印刷

ISBN 978-7-309-17161-7/R · 2070
定价:88.00 元

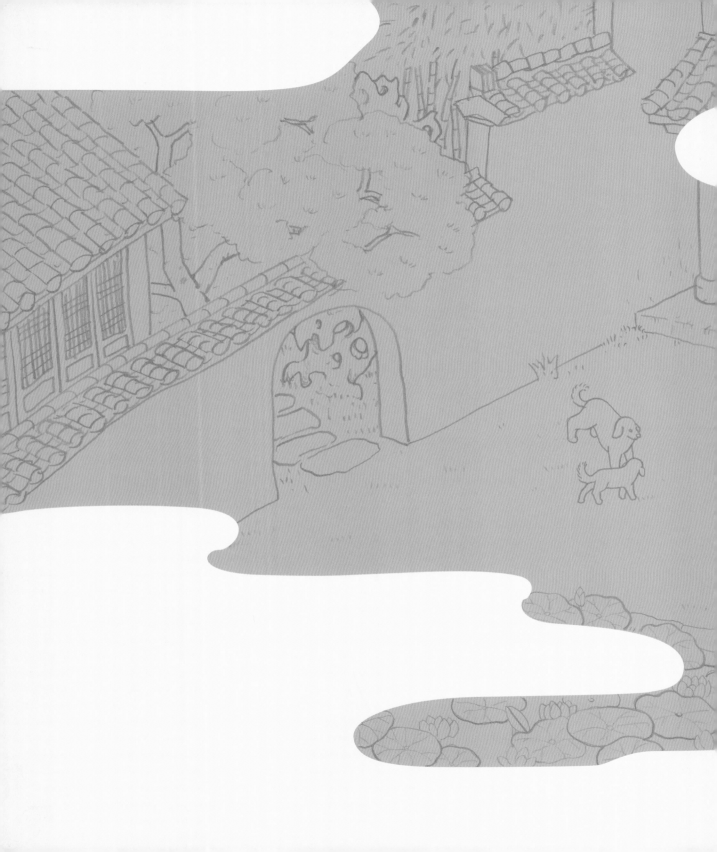